SLOW COOKER COOKBOOK FOR BEGINNERS

Effortless Cooking: Simple Recipes And Essential Tips For Delicious Slow-Cooked Meals From Breakfast To Dessert

Charlotte Harry

Table of Contents

CHAPTER ONE

INTRODUCTION TO SLOW COOKING

What Is Slow Cooking?

Slow cooking is a method of preparing food that involves cooking ingredients at a low temperature over a long period of time. This technique is typically carried out using a slow cooker or crockpot, which is an electric appliance designed to maintain a consistent low temperature, usually between 170°F and 280°F (77°C and 138°C). The primary benefit of slow cooking is the way it allows flavors to meld together and ingredients to become tender and delicious.

One of the key advantages of slow cooking is its convenience. With a slow cooker, you can set up your meal in the morning, leave it to cook throughout the day, and return home to a hot, ready-to-eat dish in the evening. This makes it an ideal cooking method for busy individuals or families who may not have the time to prepare a meal from scratch every day. The hands-off nature of slow cooking means you can focus on other tasks while your food simmers away, making it a practical solution for modern lifestyles.

The slow cooker operates by using a low, steady heat to cook food slowly and evenly. This prolonged cooking process allows tougher cuts of meat to break down and become tender, and it helps flavors develop and intensify. As a result, dishes prepared in a slow cooker often have a rich, complex taste that is difficult to achieve with other cooking methods. The low temperature also means that food is less likely to burn or overcook, providing a margin of safety for less experienced cooks.

Slow cooking is particularly well-suited for certain types of dishes, such as stews, soups, and braises. These recipes often benefit from the extended cooking time, which allows the ingredients to meld together harmoniously. Additionally, slow cookers are great for preparing one-pot meals, where all the components of the dish are cooked together, enhancing the overall flavor profile.

Another benefit of slow cooking is its ability to preserve nutrients. Since the cooking temperature is relatively low, there is less risk of nutrient loss compared to high-heat cooking methods. This makes slow-cooked meals a healthy option for those looking to maintain the nutritional integrity of their food.

Moreover, slow cooking is energy-efficient. Slow cookers use less electricity than conventional ovens, making them an environmentally friendly choice. They are also relatively inexpensive to purchase and operate, making them accessible to a wide range of households.

Benefits Of Slow Cooking

Slow cooking has gained popularity among home cooks due to its numerous benefits, transforming meal preparation into a more enjoyable and efficient process. One of the primary advantages of slow cooking is its unparalleled convenience. The method allows you to prepare your ingredients, place them in the slow cooker, set the timer, and carry on with your day. This "set it and forget it" approach is especially beneficial for busy individuals who want to enjoy a hot, home-cooked meal without dedicating hours to cooking. Whether you're at work, running errands, or simply relaxing, slow cooking ensures that dinner will be ready with minimal effort.

Another significant benefit of slow cooking is the enhancement of flavors in your dishes. The extended cooking time allows the ingredients to simmer and blend together, creating a depth of flavor that is difficult to achieve with quick-cooking methods. Spices, herbs, and other seasonings have the opportunity to infuse deeply into the food, resulting in rich, complex tastes that are often more pronounced and satisfying. This slow and gentle cooking process is ideal for dishes like stews, soups, and braises, where the flavors truly shine after hours of simmering.

Tenderness is another key advantage of slow cooking, particularly when it comes to tougher cuts of meat. Cuts like chuck roast, brisket, and pork shoulder are notoriously tough if cooked quickly, but slow cooking transforms them into tender, melt-in-your-mouth meals. The low and steady temperature breaks down the connective tissues and collagen in the meat, yielding a succulent and tender texture that is highly desirable. This method not only makes the meat more enjoyable to eat but also allows you to use more affordable cuts without sacrificing quality.

In terms of health benefits, slow cooking helps in nutrient retention, especially in vegetables. Cooking at lower temperatures helps preserve the vitamins and minerals that can be lost in high-heat cooking methods. This means that your slow-cooked meals can be both delicious and nutritious, providing you with the essential nutrients your body needs while enjoying flavorful dishes.

Lastly, slow cooking is an economical cooking method. By using less expensive cuts of meat and bulk ingredients, you can create hearty and satisfying meals without breaking the bank. Additionally, slow cookers are designed to make large quantities of food, perfect for meal prepping. You can cook in bulk, portion out the meals, and store them for later, saving both time and money in the long run. This not only reduces food waste but also ensures that you have healthy, home-cooked meals ready to go throughout the week.

Choosing The Right Slow Cooker

Choosing the right slow cooker is crucial to ensuring the best results for your slow-cooked meals. Here are several factors to consider when selecting a slow cooker:

Size: Slow cookers come in various sizes, typically ranging from 2-3 quarts to 6-8 quarts. The size you choose should depend on the number of people you're cooking for and the types of meals you plan to prepare. A smaller slow cooker, with a capacity of 2-3 quarts, is suitable for individuals or small families, making it perfect for soups, stews, or single servings. On the other hand, a larger slow cooker, around 6-8 quarts, is ideal for big batches, meal prepping, or larger families. It's especially useful when cooking whole chickens, large roasts, or preparing meals for gatherings.

Shape: Slow cookers generally come in two shapes: round and oval. Oval slow cookers tend to be more versatile as they can accommodate larger cuts of meat more easily than round ones. For example, an oval slow cooker can handle a whole chicken or a large roast without needing to cut it into smaller pieces. This shape is particularly advantageous if you frequently cook large meat portions or prefer having the flexibility to do so.

Settings: Modern slow cookers come with a variety of settings. At a minimum, look for a slow cooker that offers low, medium, and high settings, along with a warming function. The warming function keeps your food at a safe temperature after cooking is complete, ensuring that your meal stays hot without overcooking. Additionally, some models come with programmable timers that allow you to set the cooking duration. Once the time is up, these slow cookers automatically switch to the warming mode. This feature is particularly useful for busy individuals who want to set and forget their meals, ensuring that the food is ready and warm when they return home.

Features: Extra features can enhance your slow cooking experience. For instance, a locking lid is beneficial for those who frequently transport their slow cooker, as it prevents spills. A digital display can make it easier to see and set cooking times and temperatures. Removable inserts, typically made of ceramic or metal, make cleaning up much easier since you can lift the insert out and wash it separately from the heating base. Some inserts are even dishwasher safe, adding to the convenience.

Brand and Reviews: When choosing a slow cooker, consider brands that are known for their quality and reliability. Brands with a good reputation often provide better durability and customer support. Reading customer reviews can also give you valuable insights into the performance, longevity, and any potential issues of the slow cooker models you are considering. Reviews from other users can highlight the pros and cons, helping you make a more informed decision.

If you're new to slow cooking, these basic tips will help you get started and ensure your dishes turn out delicious and well-prepared.

Prep Ahead: One of the best ways to save time and streamline your slow cooking process is to prepare your ingredients the night before. This means chopping vegetables, measuring out spices, and trimming meats ahead of time. By doing this, you can simply assemble everything in the slow cooker in the morning, reducing the morning rush and making your day smoother.

Layering: Proper layering is crucial for even cooking in a slow cooker. Place denser, slower-cooking ingredients like root vegetables (e.g., carrots, potatoes, and parsnips) at the bottom of the slow cooker. These ingredients take longer to cook, and placing them at the bottom ensures they get the most heat. More delicate ingredients, such as green vegetables or fish, should be placed on top to prevent them from overcooking and becoming mushy.

Liquid Levels: Slow cookers require less liquid than traditional cooking methods because they retain moisture very effectively. Generally, aim to fill the cooker no more than two-thirds full to avoid overflow and ensure proper cooking. Too much liquid can result in a watery dish, while too little can cause ingredients to dry out. It's a delicate balance, but with practice, you'll get the hang of it.

Don't Peek: It's tempting to lift the lid and check on your meal, but each time you do, heat escapes. This loss of heat can significantly extend the cooking time and may affect the final texture and flavor of your dish. Avoid opening the lid unless absolutely necessary, especially during the first few hours of cooking when the temperature is still stabilizing.

Add Dairy Last: Ingredients like milk, cheese, and cream can curdle if cooked too long in a slow cooker. To prevent this, add dairy products during the last 30 minutes of cooking. This allows them to heat through and blend with the other ingredients without curdling or separating, ensuring a smooth and creamy consistency.

Seasoning: Slow cooking can concentrate flavors, so it's important to be cautious with seasoning. Over-seasoning at the beginning can result in an overpowering dish. It's easier to adjust the seasoning towards the end of the cooking time. Taste your dish about an hour before it's done and add more salt or spices if needed. This way, you have better control over the final flavor.

CHAPTER TWO

GETTING STARTED

Understanding Slow Cooker Settings

Slow cookers are incredibly versatile kitchen appliances that simplify meal preparation and deliver delicious, tender dishes with minimal effort. To harness their full potential, it's essential to understand the various settings most slow cookers offer: Low, High, and Keep Warm.

The Low setting is designed for long, slow cooking, typically spanning 6 to 10 hours. This gentle cooking process is perfect for tougher cuts of meat like beef brisket, pork shoulder, or lamb shanks. These meats benefit from the extended cooking time as it allows the connective tissues to break down, resulting in tender, flavorful dishes.

Stews, soups, and chili also fare well on the Low setting, as the prolonged cooking time allows flavors to meld beautifully. The Low setting is ideal for those who want to set their slow cooker in the morning and return home to a perfectly cooked meal in the evening.

In contrast, the High setting cooks food more quickly, usually within 4 to 6 hours. This setting is suitable for recipes that require less cooking time or for those occasions when you need to prepare a meal in a shorter period. While convenient, the High setting may not be ideal for all dishes. Delicate ingredients like fish, certain vegetables, and dairy products can become overcooked or lose their texture when subjected to the higher temperature. For example, a beef stew that turns out perfectly on Low might have meat that's too dry or vegetables that are too soft when cooked on High. It's essential to adjust cooking times and recipes accordingly to avoid overcooking.

The Keep Warm setting is particularly useful for maintaining the temperature of your food after it has finished cooking. This setting keeps your meal at a safe, warm temperature without continuing to cook it, ensuring your dish remains ready to serve whenever you are. It's a convenient feature for busy households, gatherings, or parties where the exact serving time might be unpredictable. You can prepare your meal ahead of time and keep it warm without compromising on quality or safety.

Modern slow cookers often come with programmable settings, adding an extra layer of convenience. These models allow you to set a specific cooking time and temperature, after which the cooker automatically switches to the Keep Warm setting. This feature is especially handy for those with hectic schedules, as it provides peace of mind that your meal will be cooked perfectly and kept warm until you're ready to eat. You can program your slow cooker in the morning, and no matter when you get home, your meal will be hot and ready to serve without the risk of overcooking.

Essential Tools And Accessories

To make the most out of your slow cooker, a few essential tools and accessories can enhance your cooking experience and ensure your meals turn out perfectly every time. These tools not only streamline your cooking process but also help in achieving the best flavors and textures in your dishes.

Firstly, a good set of measuring cups and spoons is crucial. While slow cooking is generally forgiving, accurate measurements can significantly impact the final taste of your dishes. Precise measurements ensure that the balance of flavors is just right, especially for recipes that require exact proportions of ingredients like spices and liquids. Whether you're making a hearty stew or a delicate dessert, having the right amounts can make a noticeable difference.

Next, investing in a quality cutting board and sharp knives is indispensable. Prepping your ingredients efficiently is a major part of slow cooking. A large cutting board provides ample space for chopping vegetables, slicing meats, and preparing other ingredients. Sharp knives are essential for making clean, precise cuts, which is especially important for even cooking. Dull knives can be dangerous and make the prep work unnecessarily difficult. A sharp chef's knife and a paring knife should cover most of your needs.

A ladle or a large spoon is another useful accessory for your slow cooking endeavors. Slow cookers can be quite deep, and these utensils allow you to stir and serve your dishes easily without the risk of burning yourself. A ladle is particularly handy for soups and stews, while a large spoon is great for dishing out casseroles and other chunky meals.

Heat-resistant silicone spatulas are also invaluable in a slow cooking setup. These spatulas are perfect for scraping down the sides of the slow cooker to ensure all ingredients are mixed well and nothing sticks to the sides. They can withstand high temperatures, so you don't have to worry about them melting or getting damaged.

Consider purchasing slow cooker liners for hassle-free cleanup. These disposable liners fit inside your slow cooker and can be discarded after use, saving you considerable time on washing up. They are particularly useful for recipes that tend to stick or burn, ensuring that your slow cooker remains clean and ready for the next use.

Lastly, a good set of oven mitts is essential for safely handling the hot slow cooker insert. Slow cookers can get very hot, and having reliable oven mitts protects your hands and arms from burns when you need to lift the insert out of the cooker, stir the contents, or serve the food.

Slow Cooking Do's And Don'ts

Slow cooking can be a game-changer in your kitchen, making it easy to create delicious, tender meals with minimal effort. However, there are some essential do's and don'ts to ensure your slow-cooked dishes turn out perfectly every time. Here's a guide to help you get the best results.

Do's:

1. Use the Right Cut of Meat:

Selecting the appropriate cut of meat is crucial for successful slow cooking. Tougher cuts, such as chuck roast, brisket, and pork shoulder, are ideal because they break down and become tender over long, slow cooking times. These cuts are often more flavorful and economical, making them perfect for slow cooker recipes.

2. Brown Your Meat First:

While it's not always necessary, browning your meat in a skillet before adding it to the slow cooker can significantly enhance the flavor of your dish. The caramelization that occurs during browning adds depth and complexity to the final meal.

3. Layer Your Ingredients Correctly:

Proper layering of ingredients is essential for even cooking. Place root vegetables like potatoes and carrots at the bottom of the slow cooker, as they take longer to cook. Next, add the meat, and finally, pour in any liquids. This arrangement ensures that everything cooks evenly and is perfectly done at the same time.

4. Keep the Lid Closed:

It can be tempting to lift the lid and check on your meal, but every time you do, heat escapes, and the cooking time extends. Only open the lid if absolutely necessary, such as to add ingredients that need less cooking time.

Don'ts:

1. Don't Overfill Your Slow Cooker:

Avoid filling your slow cooker more than two-thirds full. Overfilling can lead to uneven cooking and spills. If your slow cooker is too full, the heat may not circulate properly, and your food may not cook as intended.

2. Don't Add Dairy Products Too Early:

Dairy products like milk, cheese, and cream can curdle if cooked too long in a slow cooker. To prevent this, add these ingredients during the last 30 minutes of cooking. This step ensures they integrate well without affecting the texture of your dish.

3. Don't Forget to Season Properly:

Slow cooking can sometimes mute flavors, so it's important to taste and adjust seasonings before serving. Don't hesitate to add a bit more salt, pepper, or herbs towards the end of the cooking time to ensure your meal is flavorful.

4. Don't Use Frozen Ingredients:

Adding frozen meat or vegetables can lower the temperature in the slow cooker, affecting the cooking time and potentially leading to food safety issues. Always thaw ingredients first to maintain a consistent cooking temperature and ensure your dish cooks evenly.

Prepping Ingredients

Prepping ingredients is a crucial step in slow cooking that sets the foundation for a successful and flavorful dish. Start by thoroughly washing and chopping your vegetables. Since slow cooking enhances the natural sweetness of vegetables, it's important to cut them into uniform pieces. This ensures even cooking and a consistent texture throughout your dish. Pay particular attention to root vegetables like carrots and potatoes, which can take longer to cook. Cutting them into smaller, uniform pieces will help them cook at the same rate as other ingredients.

For meats, trimming excess fat is essential. Slow cooking can render fat effectively, but too much can make your dish overly greasy. By trimming the fat, you ensure a leaner, healthier meal without sacrificing flavor. If you have the time, consider marinating your meats overnight. A simple marinade using oil, vinegar, herbs, and spices can add an extra depth of flavor that penetrates the meat as it cooks slowly. Just remember to shake off any excess marinade before placing the meat in the slow cooker to avoid diluting the dish's overall flavor.

When a recipe calls for sautéing onions or garlic, do this step before adding them to the slow cooker. Sautéing these aromatics releases their natural sweetness and intensifies their flavors, contributing to a richer, more complex taste in the final dish. This small extra step can make a significant difference in the overall flavor profile of your meal.

Measuring out your liquids carefully is another important aspect of prepping for slow cooking. Whether you're using broth, wine, or water, the right amount of liquid is crucial. Slow cookers require less liquid than traditional cooking methods because they create steam and trap moisture, preventing the dish from drying out. Even if it seems like there's not enough liquid at the beginning, resist the urge to add more. Too much liquid can result in a watery dish, diluting the flavors. Instead, trust the process; the steam and moisture will ensure your meal stays moist and flavorful.

By taking the time to properly prep your ingredients—washing and chopping vegetables uniformly, trimming excess fat from meats, marinating if possible, sautéing aromatics, and measuring liquids accurately—you set yourself up for slow cooking success. These steps may seem simple, but they are fundamental to achieving the rich, deep flavors that make slow-cooked meals so satisfying. Preparing with care ensures that each ingredient contributes its best to the final dish, resulting in a meal that is both delicious and perfectly cooked.

CHAPTER THREE

BREAKFAST DELIGHTS

Overnight Oats And Porridges

Overnight oats and porridges are an excellent way to start your day, offering a blend of convenience, nutrition, and deliciousness. They are incredibly easy to prepare and can be customized to suit your taste preferences, making them a versatile option for busy mornings.

Overnight Oats

Overnight oats require no cooking and are perfect for those who need a quick, grab-and-go breakfast. The basic concept is to soak oats in a liquid of your choice overnight, allowing them to absorb the liquid and soften. By morning, you have a ready-to-eat meal that's both nutritious and satisfying.

To prepare overnight oats, start by combining rolled oats with your preferred liquid. Options include regular milk, almond milk, soy milk, or even yogurt. This provides a creamy base that complements the oats' texture. For flavor, consider adding a sweetener such as honey, maple syrup, or vanilla extract. You can also enhance the nutritional value by mixing in fruits and nuts. Popular choices include berries, bananas, apples, chia seeds, flaxseeds, and almonds. These additions not only boost the nutritional profile but also add delightful textures and flavors.

Mix all the ingredients in a bowl or jar, ensuring everything is well combined. Cover the container and refrigerate it overnight. The oats will absorb the liquid and flavors, resulting in a creamy, delicious breakfast by morning. When you're ready to eat, give the mixture a good stir, and you can enjoy it cold or warm it up slightly if you prefer.

Porridges

Porridges offer a warm, comforting alternative to overnight oats. They are typically cooked, but you can also prepare them in a slow cooker for a hands-off approach. This method is perfect for those who enjoy a hot breakfast without the morning hassle.

To make porridge, steel-cut oats are an excellent choice due to their hearty texture. Combine the oats with water or milk, a pinch of salt, and your favorite flavorings in a slow cooker. Popular flavorings include cinnamon, nutmeg, and vanilla. Set the slow cooker to low and let it cook overnight. By morning, you'll have a pot of warm, creamy porridge ready to eat.

In the morning, give the porridge a good stir to achieve a uniform consistency. Serve it in bowls and add your desired toppings. Fresh fruits like berries, sliced bananas, and chopped apples work wonderfully. Nuts, seeds, and a drizzle of honey or maple syrup can also enhance the flavor and nutritional value.

Breakfast Casseroles

Breakfast casseroles are a fantastic option for a delicious and convenient morning meal. They are perfect for feeding a crowd or preparing ahead of time, ensuring you have a hearty breakfast ready for the week. Utilizing a slow cooker can simplify the process even further, allowing you to assemble the casserole the night before and let it cook overnight, so it's hot and ready when you wake up.

To begin, choose a base for your casserole. Popular options include bread cubes, hash browns, or cooked grains like quinoa. These bases provide a satisfying texture and absorb the flavors of the other ingredients. Next, add layers of vegetables. Spinach, bell peppers, and onions are excellent choices, offering a variety of colors, textures, and nutrients. Including proteins is essential for a well-rounded meal. Sausage, bacon, or beans can add savory flavors and protein to keep you full throughout the morning.

The heart of the casserole is the egg mixture. Whisk together eggs, milk, and your choice of seasonings. Common seasonings include salt, pepper, garlic powder, and herbs like parsley or chives. The egg mixture binds the ingredients together and creates a cohesive dish. Pour the mixture over the layered ingredients in the slow cooker, ensuring everything is evenly covered. Cover and cook on low for 6-8 hours. The slow cooking process allows the flavors to meld and the eggs to set, resulting in a perfectly cooked casserole.

If you prefer a sweeter start to your day, consider making a sweet breakfast casserole. This variation uses bread, eggs, milk, and sweet additions like cinnamon, sugar, and fruit. This can be a delightful alternative to traditional French toast. Begin with a base of bread cubes, then add your favorite fruits. Apples, berries, and bananas work particularly well. Whisk together eggs, milk, cinnamon, and sugar, and pour the mixture over the bread and fruit. Cook in the slow cooker until the eggs are set and the casserole is firm.

Sweet breakfast casseroles can be served with a drizzle of maple syrup or a sprinkle of powdered sugar for an extra touch of sweetness. They are perfect for special occasions or a weekend treat, providing a warm and comforting meal that feels indulgent yet is easy to prepare.

Egg Dishes

Egg dishes are incredibly versatile and can be easily made in a slow cooker, offering a convenient way to prepare breakfast or brunch. Whether you prefer frittatas, quiches, or simple scrambled eggs, the slow cooker can handle it all, providing delicious and effortless meals.

To make a slow cooker frittata, start by whisking together eggs, milk, cheese, and your favorite fillings such as vegetables, meats, and herbs. Common fillings include spinach, bell peppers, mushrooms, onions, ham, bacon, or sausage. Pour the mixture into the slow cooker, cover, and cook on low for 2-3 hours or until the eggs are set and cooked through. The slow cooker frittata is perfect for a protein-packed breakfast and can be customized to include whatever ingredients you have on hand, making it a great option for using up leftovers. It's also an excellent dish for entertaining guests, as it can be prepared ahead of time and left to cook while you attend to other tasks.

Another fantastic option is to make a breakfast burrito filling in the slow cooker.

Combine eggs, cheese, cooked sausage or bacon, and vegetables like diced tomatoes, onions, and bell peppers in the slow cooker. Cook on low for a few hours, stirring occasionally until the eggs are cooked and the mixture is well combined. This filling can then be served in tortillas for quick and easy breakfast burritos. It's a convenient way to prepare breakfast for a crowd or to have ready-made burrito fillings that can be reheated for a fast weekday breakfast.

Scrambled eggs can also be made in the slow cooker, which is particularly useful for cooking a large batch without having to stand over the stove. To make slow cooker scrambled eggs, simply whisk the eggs with milk and seasonings like salt, pepper, and any herbs or spices you prefer. Pour the mixture into the slow cooker and cook on low, stirring occasionally until the eggs are cooked through. This method ensures evenly cooked scrambled eggs and frees you up to prepare other parts of your meal.

The slow cooker method for egg dishes not only simplifies the cooking process but also produces consistently delicious results. Whether you're making a hearty frittata, a versatile breakfast burrito filling, or perfectly cooked scrambled eggs, the slow cooker offers a hands-off approach that can save time and effort. These dishes are perfect for busy mornings, family gatherings, or meal prep, ensuring you have a nutritious and satisfying breakfast with minimal hassle.

Slow Cooker Bread And Muffins

Baking bread and muffins in a slow cooker might sound unusual, but it's a convenient and practical way to make fresh baked goods without the need for an oven. The slow cooker creates a moist environment that is ideal for baking, making it a versatile tool in the kitchen.

To bake bread in a slow cooker, start by preparing your dough as you normally would. This includes mixing the ingredients, kneading the dough, and allowing it to rise if necessary. Once your dough is ready, line the slow cooker with parchment paper. This prevents the dough from sticking and makes for easier cleanup. Place the dough in the slow cooker, cover it with the lid, and set the cooker to high. The bread should cook for approximately 2-3 hours. The exact time will depend on the size and type of bread you're making. You'll know it's done when the bread is cooked through and has a golden crust. One of the great things about using a slow cooker for bread is that it works well with a variety of bread types. Whether you're making yeast breads, quick breads, or even sweet treats like cinnamon rolls, the slow cooker can handle it all.

Muffins are another baked good that can be easily made in a slow cooker. For this, you can use silicone muffin cups or line the slow cooker with parchment paper. Silicone cups are especially useful because they are reusable and make for easy removal of the muffins once they are cooked. Prepare your muffin batter as usual, and fill the cups about two-thirds full. Place the filled cups in the slow cooker, cover it with the lid, and set the cooker to high. The muffins will take about 1-2 hours to cook. Again, the exact time will depend on the size and type of muffins you are making. To check if they are done, insert a toothpick into the center of a muffin; if it comes out clean, the muffins are ready.

Using a slow cooker for baking has several advantages. Firstly, it doesn't heat up the kitchen, which is a great benefit during hot weather. Secondly, it allows you to bake without the need for an oven, making it perfect for those who might not have access to a full kitchen. Lastly, the slow, steady heat of the slow cooker can result in baked goods that are exceptionally moist and tender.

CHAPTER FOUR

SOUPS AND STEWS

Hearty Vegetable Soups

Hearty vegetable soups are an excellent way to pack a variety of fresh produce into your meals, offering nourishment and satisfaction in each bowl. These soups are not only comforting but also incredibly versatile, allowing you to use whatever vegetables you have on hand. This flexibility makes them an ideal choice for a nutritious meal that can be adapted to the seasons or your personal preferences.

To start your soup, begin with a flavorful base. Sautéing onions, garlic, and celery in a large pot sets the foundation for a rich taste. These aromatic ingredients release their flavors, creating a savory backdrop for the rest of your vegetables. Once they are softened and fragrant, it's time to add the other ingredients.

Diced tomatoes are a fantastic addition, providing acidity and a slight sweetness that balances the soup. Carrots and potatoes contribute heartiness and texture, making the soup filling. Leafy greens, such as spinach or kale, can be added for an additional nutrient boost, bringing in vitamins and minerals that are essential for overall health. Don't hesitate to incorporate other vegetables you enjoy or need to use up—zucchini, bell peppers, and green beans are all great options.

When it comes to seasoning, herbs play a crucial role in enhancing the flavors of your soup. Dried or fresh herbs like thyme, oregano, and basil add depth and complexity. Feel free to experiment with spices as well; a pinch of red pepper flakes can introduce a gentle heat, while a dash of smoked paprika can provide a unique twist.

The cooking process is straightforward. After sautéing your base vegetables, stir in the remaining ingredients along with vegetable broth to create a comforting and nourishing broth. Allow the soup to simmer for about 30 minutes, which will give the vegetables time to soften and the flavors to meld beautifully. Keep an eye on the texture of the vegetables, ensuring they are tender but not mushy.

Meat-Based Stews

As the weather cools down, there's nothing quite like a hearty meat-based stew to warm your soul and satisfy your hunger. These comforting dishes are not only delicious but also versatile, allowing you to experiment with different meats and vegetables to create a unique flavor experience each time.

Classic meat-based stews often feature beef, chicken, or lamb, each bringing its own distinct taste and texture to the dish. Beef stew, for instance, is rich and robust, often enhanced with ingredients like red wine or stout for added depth. Chicken stew, on the other hand, is lighter and can be flavored with herbs such as thyme and rosemary, while lamb stew tends to be aromatic and tender, often featuring spices like cumin and coriander.

The key to a great stew begins with the browning of the meat. Start by cutting your chosen meat into large chunks, ensuring they are of uniform size for even cooking.

Heat a heavy pot or Dutch oven over medium-high heat and add a bit of oil. Once the oil is shimmering, add the meat in batches, being careful not to overcrowd the pot. This browning process caramelizes the surface of the meat, creating a rich, savory flavor that enhances the entire dish.

After the meat is nicely browned, remove it from the pot and set it aside. In the same pot, add chopped onions and minced garlic, sautéing until they become fragrant and translucent. This step adds a foundational layer of flavor to the stew. Next, introduce your choice of vegetables—carrots, potatoes, celery, and bell peppers work wonderfully. Sauté these ingredients until they start to soften, which usually takes about five to seven minutes.

Once your vegetables are ready, return the browned meat to the pot. Pour in enough broth (beef, chicken, or vegetable) to cover the ingredients, and add your preferred seasonings—think bay leaves, black pepper, or a pinch of paprika for warmth. Bring the mixture to a gentle boil, then reduce the heat to low. Cover the pot and let it simmer for at least one to two hours, or until the meat is fork-tender and the flavors have melded beautifully.

The final result is a hearty stew that is perfect for serving over a bed of fluffy rice or alongside crusty bread, allowing you to soak up every drop of the savory broth. Whether enjoyed on a chilly evening or shared with family and friends, a meat-based stew is a timeless dish that never fails to comfort and delight.

Creamy soups and chowders bring a delightful richness to the table, making them an ideal choice for those moments when you crave something indulgent and satisfying. Their velvety texture and robust flavors create a comforting experience, perfect for warming up on chilly days or impressing guests with a touch of culinary flair.

To begin crafting your creamy soup or chowder, start by sautéing a base of finely chopped onions and minced garlic in a generous splash of olive oil or butter. This aromatic foundation sets the stage for the deliciousness to come. As the onions become translucent and fragrant, it's time to add in diced potatoes. Potatoes not only contribute to the creaminess of the final dish but also provide substance, making the soup hearty.

Next, incorporate your choice of vegetables. For classic chowder, sweet corn and tender clams are traditional favorites. If you prefer a vegetarian option, consider using seasonal vegetables like carrots, celery, or bell peppers, which add flavor and color. As the vegetables cook, they will become tender and infuse the broth with their natural sweetness.

Once the vegetables are sufficiently softened, it's time to elevate the dish with cream or a dairy alternative, such as coconut milk or cashew cream. Stir this in gently, allowing the mixture to become luxuriously creamy. For seafood chowders, a dash of Old Bay seasoning or a sprinkle of smoked paprika adds depth and a touch of spice, enhancing the overall flavor profile.

After adding the cream, let the soup simmer gently. This step is crucial for allowing the flavors to meld beautifully, creating a harmonious blend that tantalizes the taste buds. Depending on your texture preference, you can use an immersion blender to achieve a smooth, velvety consistency or leave it chunky for a heartier feel.

Serving is where you can truly make your creamy soup shine. Consider garnishing with a sprinkle of fresh herbs like chives, parsley, or dill, which not only add vibrant color but also a fresh burst of flavor. For added texture, a handful of homemade croutons or a drizzle of flavored oil can take your soup to the next level.

International Soup Recipes

Exploring international soups can add excitement and variety to your meal planning, allowing you to experience different cultures through their culinary traditions. Each region has its unique take on soup, showcasing local ingredients and flavors. From the spicy Tom Yum of Thailand to the hearty Minestrone of Italy, these dishes offer a delightful way to warm up and nourish the soul.

To start your culinary journey in Asia, consider making Pho, a traditional Vietnamese soup that features a fragrant broth, rice noodles, and fresh herbs. The heart of Pho lies in its broth, which requires hours of simmering to achieve a deep, rich flavor. Begin with beef bones or chicken, adding spices like star anise, cinnamon, and cloves to infuse the broth with aromatic notes. Once the broth is ready, serve it over rice noodles and top with thinly sliced beef or chicken, along with fresh herbs like basil and cilantro. A squeeze of lime and slices of jalapeño add a refreshing kick, making this soup not just delicious but also a vibrant meal.

Moving west to Italy, Minestrone is a beloved classic that showcases the bounty of seasonal vegetables. This thick, hearty soup typically includes ingredients such as beans, pasta, and whatever vegetables are at their peak, from zucchini to carrots and tomatoes. The beauty of Minestrone lies in its versatility; you can adapt the recipe based on what's available in your pantry or what's in season at your local market. Start by sautéing onions, garlic, and celery in olive oil, then add your chosen vegetables, beans, and vegetable or chicken broth. Let it simmer until everything is tender, and finish with a sprinkle of Parmesan cheese for an extra layer of flavor.

For a Middle Eastern twist, try making Lentil Soup, a nutritious and satisfying option that is perfect for cozy evenings. This soup is flavored with warming spices such as cumin and coriander, along with a hint of lemon juice for brightness. Begin by sautéing onions and garlic in olive oil, then add lentils, diced tomatoes, and spices. Simmer until the lentils are tender, and finish with a squeeze of lemon for a refreshing contrast to the earthy lentils. This soup not only warms you up but is also packed with protein and fiber, making it a healthy choice.

CHAPTER FIVE

MAIN COURSES

Chicken And Poultry Dishes

Slow cookers are an ideal kitchen appliance for preparing chicken and other poultry dishes, offering the convenience of achieving tender, juicy results with minimal effort. One classic recipe that exemplifies this is Slow Cooker Chicken Curry. This dish is not only flavorful but also simple to prepare. To start, gather your ingredients: chicken thighs, diced onions, garlic, ginger, coconut milk, and a selection of curry spices such as turmeric, cumin, coriander, and garam masala. Begin by placing the chicken thighs at the bottom of the slow cooker. Next, add the diced onions, minced garlic, and freshly grated ginger on top of the chicken. Pour in the coconut milk, ensuring that the chicken and other ingredients are well-coated. Finally, sprinkle the curry spices evenly over the mixture. Set the slow cooker to low and allow it to cook for 6-8 hours. During this time, the flavors will meld together, and the chicken will become incredibly tender. By the end of the cooking period, you will have a rich, aromatic chicken curry that is perfect for serving with rice or naan bread.

Another beloved poultry dish for the slow cooker is Slow Cooker BBQ Chicken. This recipe is particularly appealing for its simplicity and the tangy, satisfying flavor it delivers. To make this dish, you will need chicken breasts, your favorite barbecue sauce, and a splash of apple cider vinegar. Start by placing the chicken breasts in the slow cooker. In a separate bowl, mix the barbecue sauce with the apple cider vinegar to add a bit of tanginess to the dish. Pour this mixture over the chicken breasts, ensuring they are fully coated. Set the slow cooker to low and cook for 6-7 hours. During this time, the chicken will absorb the barbecue sauce, becoming tender and infused with flavor. Once the cooking time is up, use two forks to shred the chicken directly in the slow cooker. The shredded chicken can be used as a delicious filling for sandwiches, wraps, or even served over a salad for a lighter option.

Both of these recipes highlight the versatility and convenience of using a slow cooker for poultry dishes. The Slow Cooker Chicken Curry offers a rich, aromatic experience with its blend of spices and creamy coconut milk, while the Slow Cooker BBQ Chicken provides a tangy, savory option perfect for casual meals. These dishes not only save time and effort but also ensure that you can enjoy flavorful, home-cooked meals with ease. Whether you are preparing a comforting curry or a tangy barbecue chicken, the slow cooker proves to be an invaluable tool in creating delicious and effortless meals.

Beef And Pork Recipes

For beef lovers, a slow cooker beef stew can be a comforting and hearty meal. Begin by selecting quality chunks of beef and browning them in a skillet. This initial step enhances the flavor by creating a rich, caramelized crust on the meat. Once browned, transfer the beef to your slow cooker. Next, prepare the vegetables. Peel and chop carrots and potatoes into bite-sized pieces, ensuring they are uniform in size for even cooking. Dice an onion and mince a few cloves of garlic. These aromatics will add depth to your stew.

Add the vegetables to the slow cooker, layering them over the beef. Pour in beef broth until the ingredients are almost submerged. The broth will blend with the juices from the meat and vegetables, creating a flavorful base. For seasoning, add a few sprigs of fresh thyme and a couple of bay leaves. These herbs will infuse the stew with their earthy and slightly minty flavors as it cooks. Set your slow cooker to low and let the stew simmer gently for 8-10 hours. This slow cooking process will tenderize the beef, allowing the flavors to meld together beautifully. By the end of the cooking time, you will have a delicious, hearty beef stew perfect for a comforting dinner.

If pork is your choice, slow cooker pulled pork is a crowd-pleaser that is both simple to prepare and versatile. Start with a pork shoulder, also known as pork butt, which is well-marbled and ideal for slow cooking. Create a spice rub using a blend of your favorite spices. Common choices include paprika, cumin, garlic powder, onion powder, salt, and pepper. Rub the spice mixture generously all over the pork shoulder, ensuring it is well coated.

Place the seasoned pork shoulder into the slow cooker. Add sliced onions on top and around the meat. These onions will cook down and add a sweet, savory flavor to the pork. Pour in a bit of broth to keep the meat moist during cooking. Set the slow cooker to low and cook for 8-10 hours. The slow, gentle heat will break down the pork fibers, resulting in tender, succulent meat that can be easily shredded with a fork.

Once the pork is done, remove it from the slow cooker and shred it using two forks. Mix the shredded pork with your favorite barbecue sauce for added flavor. This pulled pork is incredibly versatile. Serve it on buns for sandwiches, use it as a filling for tacos, or enjoy it on its own with a side of coleslaw. Slow cooker pulled pork is a dish that is sure to satisfy any crowd, making it a perfect choice for gatherings or family dinners.

Vegetarian And Vegan Main Courses

Vegetarian and vegan meals are incredibly satisfying and flavorful, especially when prepared in a slow cooker. The beauty of these meals lies in their simplicity and the way the slow cooking process melds flavors together, creating hearty and nutritious dishes that are perfect for meal prep. Here, we explore two delightful recipes: Slow Cooker Lentil Soup and Slow Cooker Ratatouille.

Slow Cooker Lentil Soup

Lentil soup is a classic comfort food that is both nourishing and delicious. To prepare this in a slow cooker, you will need the following ingredients: lentils, diced tomatoes, carrots, celery, onions, garlic, and vegetable broth. Begin by rinsing the lentils under cold water to remove any debris. Next, chop the carrots, celery, and onions into bite-sized pieces. Mince the garlic cloves.

Place the lentils, diced tomatoes, carrots, celery, onions, and garlic into the slow cooker. Pour in the vegetable broth, ensuring that all ingredients are well submerged. Season the mixture with your choice of herbs and spices. Common seasonings for lentil soup include bay leaves, thyme, cumin, and paprika. A pinch of salt and pepper can also enhance the flavor.

Set the slow cooker on low and let it cook for 6-8 hours. During this time, the lentils will become tender, and the vegetables will soften, releasing their natural flavors into the broth. The result is a rich, hearty soup that is perfect for a cozy meal. Slow Cooker Lentil Soup is not only nutritious but also versatile; you can add spinach or kale towards the end of the cooking process for an extra boost of greens.

Slow Cooker Ratatouille

Ratatouille is a vibrant, vegetable-packed dish that showcases the best of Mediterranean flavors. To make this in a slow cooker, you will need zucchini, eggplant, bell peppers, tomatoes, garlic, olive oil, and a selection of herbs such as basil and oregano.

Start by slicing the zucchini, eggplant, and bell peppers into even, thin rounds. Core and chop the tomatoes. Mince the garlic. In the slow cooker, begin layering the vegetables in an alternating pattern, creating a visually appealing arrangement. Drizzle olive oil over the layered vegetables, ensuring an even coating. Sprinkle minced garlic and dried herbs over the top, adding a touch of salt and pepper to taste.

Set the slow cooker on low and cook for 6-8 hours. The slow cooking process allows the vegetables to become tender while maintaining their shape, and the flavors meld together beautifully. The garlic and herbs infuse the dish with a fragrant aroma and delicious taste.

Slow Cooker Ratatouille is a versatile dish that can be enjoyed in various ways. Serve it with crusty bread for a rustic meal, or spoon it over pasta or rice for a heartier option. This dish is not only flavorful but also packed with vitamins and minerals, making it a healthy choice for any meal.

Seafood Delights

When it comes to slow cooking, most people instinctively think of hearty meats and robust stews. However, seafood can be an unexpected but delightful star in slow cooker recipes, providing a fresh and flavorful twist. Two standout dishes that showcase the versatility of seafood in slow cookers are Slow Cooker Lemon Garlic Shrimp and Slow Cooker Fish Tacos.

Slow Cooker Lemon Garlic Shrimp is an effortless and delicious option for seafood lovers. Begin by gathering your ingredients: fresh shrimp, minced garlic, lemon juice, olive oil, and your choice of herbs such as parsley or thyme. The preparation is straightforward—toss the shrimp with the minced garlic, a generous squeeze of lemon juice, a drizzle of olive oil, and the herbs. Mix everything well to ensure the shrimp is evenly coated. Place the seasoned shrimp in the slow cooker and set it to low. Cook for 1 to 2 hours, keeping a close eye on the shrimp to avoid overcooking. Overcooked shrimp can become tough and chewy, so it's important to check them periodically for doneness. Once the shrimp are tender and cooked through, they are ready to serve. This dish pairs beautifully with a variety of sides. For a light and refreshing meal, serve the lemon garlic shrimp over a bed of pasta tossed with a bit of olive oil and fresh herbs, or accompany it with a crisp, fresh salad.

For a more substantial seafood dish, Slow Cooker Fish Tacos are an excellent choice. Begin by selecting white fish fillets such as tilapia, cod, or halibut. Place the fillets in the slow cooker along with diced tomatoes, fresh lime juice, and a blend of your favorite spices—cumin, chili powder, and garlic powder work particularly well. Set the slow cooker to low and cook for 2 to 3 hours. The slow cooking process allows the flavors to meld beautifully, infusing the fish with a rich, tangy taste. Once the fish is cooked through and flakes easily with a fork, it's ready to be transformed into tacos.

To assemble the tacos, flake the fish into bite-sized pieces and place them in warm corn tortillas. Top with creamy slices of avocado, crunchy shredded cabbage, and a dollop of fresh salsa. The result is a vibrant and satisfying meal that's perfect for a casual dinner or a fun gathering with friends.

CHAPTER SIX

SIDE DISHES

Vegetable Sides

Vegetable side dishes play a vital role in enhancing the flavor and nutritional value of any meal. They can vary from simple preparations like steamed vegetables to more intricate dishes. A popular choice for vegetable sides is roasted vegetables. This method typically involves a combination of carrots, bell peppers, zucchini, and onions. By tossing these vegetables with olive oil, salt, pepper, and a selection of your preferred herbs, and then roasting them in the oven, you can enhance their natural sweetness and achieve a delightful texture that complements any main course.

Roasted vegetables are not only delicious but also highly versatile. You can experiment with different vegetables depending on what is in season or available. For instance, adding root vegetables like sweet potatoes or parsnips can provide additional layers of flavor and a heartier texture. The key is to ensure that all the vegetables are cut to a uniform size to ensure even cooking. Roasting at a high temperature, typically around 425°F (220°C), helps to caramelize the natural sugars in the vegetables, resulting in a deep, rich flavor.

Another fantastic vegetable side dish is sautéed spinach or kale. This quick and straightforward dish requires only a few ingredients but delivers a powerful flavor punch. Start by heating a little olive oil in a pan over medium-high heat. Add garlic and sauté until it becomes fragrant. Then, add the spinach or kale and cook until the greens are wilted and tender. This process usually takes just a few minutes. To elevate the dish, you can add a squeeze of lemon juice, which brightens the flavors, and a sprinkle of red pepper flakes for a hint of heat. This side dish is not only flavorful but also packed with nutrients, making it a great addition to any meal.

Steamed vegetables like broccoli or green beans are also excellent options for side dishes. Steaming is a gentle cooking method that helps retain the vegetables' nutrients and vibrant colors. To prepare, simply steam the broccoli or green beans until they are tender yet still crisp. Once steamed, you can enhance the flavor by drizzling a bit of olive oil over the vegetables and seasoning them with a pinch of salt and a dash of black pepper. This simple preparation allows the natural flavors of the vegetables to shine through.

Rice And Grain Dishes

Rice and grain dishes make wonderful side dishes that can complement a wide variety of main courses. One classic choice is pilaf, a dish that brings together the simplicity of rice with the rich flavors of onions, garlic, and broth. Pilaf is a versatile dish, often enjoyed for its fluffy texture and the depth of flavor it acquires from the cooking process. To make pilaf, start by sautéing finely chopped onions and garlic in a bit of olive oil until they are soft and aromatic. Next, add the rice, stirring to coat each grain with the oil and allowing it to toast slightly. Pour in a savory broth, whether chicken, vegetable, or beef, and bring the mixture to a boil before reducing the heat to a simmer. Cover the pot and let the rice cook until all the liquid is absorbed, resulting in a flavorful and fluffy dish.

To elevate the basic pilaf, consider adding a variety of vegetables and other ingredients. Peas, carrots, and bell peppers can be stirred in during the cooking process, adding both color and nutritional value. For a touch of crunch and sweetness, toasted nuts such as almonds or cashews and dried fruits like raisins or apricots can be mixed in. These additions not only enhance the taste but also provide interesting textures that make the dish more satisfying.

Quinoa, a nutrient-rich grain, is another excellent option for creating versatile and healthy side dishes. Known for its high protein content and fluffy texture, quinoa can be cooked similarly to rice, in vegetable or chicken broth, to infuse it with flavor. Once cooked, it can serve as the base for a refreshing quinoa salad. Combine the quinoa with chopped fresh herbs like parsley or cilantro, diced tomatoes, cucumbers, and a simple vinaigrette made from olive oil, lemon juice, salt, and pepper. This salad is light, nutritious, and perfect for pairing with a variety of main courses, from grilled chicken to roasted vegetables.

Couscous, a staple in North African cuisine, is another grain that is quick and easy to prepare. Its tiny, pasta-like grains cook rapidly, making it an ideal choice for a last-minute side dish. To prepare couscous, simply pour boiling water or broth over it, cover, and let it steam for a few minutes. Once it has absorbed all the liquid, fluff it with a fork to separate the grains. For added flavor, mix in sautéed onions, raisins, and chopped parsley. The sweetness of the raisins contrasts beautifully with the savory onions, creating a dish that is both aromatic and flavorful.

Slow Cooker Beans And Lentils

Beans and lentils, when cooked in a slow cooker, transform into hearty and nutritious side dishes that can complement any meal. The slow cooking method is particularly effective for these legumes, as it allows them to become tender while absorbing all the rich and varied flavors of the accompanying ingredients.

Slow-Cooked Baked Beans

A classic recipe that showcases the versatility and deliciousness of slow-cooked beans is slow-cooked baked beans. To prepare this dish, begin by soaking dried beans overnight. This step is crucial as it helps to soften the beans, making them easier to cook and digest. After soaking, drain and rinse the beans before adding them to the slow cooker.

The base of the slow-cooked baked beans typically includes tomato sauce, which provides a tangy and rich flavor. To enhance the taste, add ingredients like molasses, mustard, and brown sugar. Molasses gives the beans a deep, slightly sweet flavor, while mustard adds a hint of sharpness. Brown sugar not only sweetens the dish but also helps to create a thick, caramelized sauce that coats the beans beautifully.

As the beans cook slowly over several hours, they absorb the flavors of these ingredients, becoming incredibly tender and flavorful. This method of cooking allows the beans to break down gradually, resulting in a dish with a perfect texture and a rich, savory taste.

Lentil Stew

Lentils are another excellent option for the slow cooker. A simple yet delicious lentil stew can be made by combining lentils with diced tomatoes, onions, garlic, carrots, and vegetable broth. The key to a great lentil stew is to allow it to cook on low heat for several hours. This slow cooking process helps the lentils to soften and absorb the flavors of the vegetables and broth, creating a dish that is both hearty and comforting.

For a more aromatic and flavorful lentil stew, consider adding spices such as cumin, coriander, and turmeric. Cumin and coriander provide a warm, earthy flavor, while turmeric adds a vibrant color and a subtle hint of bitterness. These spices not only enhance the taste of the lentils but also offer various health benefits, making the dish even more nutritious.

Another variation of lentil stew is to incorporate different types of vegetables and herbs. Adding leafy greens like spinach or kale towards the end of the cooking process can boost the nutritional value and add a fresh, slightly bitter taste that balances the richness of the stew. Fresh herbs like parsley or cilantro can be sprinkled on top before serving to add a burst of color and flavor.

Sauces And Gravies

Sauces and gravies are the perfect finishing touch for many side dishes, adding richness and depth of flavor. They can elevate a simple dish to something extraordinary with their complex and complementary tastes. One classic sauce is a simple tomato sauce, a staple in many cuisines. To create this sauce, start by sautéing finely chopped onions and minced garlic in a generous amount of olive oil until they become fragrant and translucent. This forms the aromatic base of the sauce. Then, add a can of crushed tomatoes, ensuring they are of good quality for the best flavor. Season the mixture with salt, freshly ground black pepper, and a pinch of sugar to balance the acidity of the tomatoes. Allow the sauce to simmer gently over low heat, stirring occasionally, until it thickens and the flavors meld together. This simple tomato sauce can be used in a variety of dishes, from topping al dente pasta and fluffy rice to enhancing the flavors of roasted vegetables.

A creamy mushroom gravy is another excellent option that brings a rich, savory element to side dishes. Begin by sautéing sliced mushrooms in a generous amount of butter over medium heat. Cook the mushrooms until they are golden brown and tender, releasing their juices and developing a deep, earthy flavor. Once the mushrooms are cooked, sprinkle in some all-purpose flour to create a roux. Stir the flour and mushrooms together until the flour is fully incorporated and starts to turn a light golden color. Gradually whisk in vegetable or chicken broth, allowing the mixture to come to a gentle simmer. As the gravy thickens, add a splash of heavy cream to create a smooth and velvety texture. Season the gravy with salt, black pepper, and a touch of thyme or rosemary to enhance the mushroom's natural flavors. This creamy mushroom gravy pairs wonderfully with mashed potatoes, roasted meats, or even drizzled over savory biscuits.

For a lighter, fresher option, consider making a lemon herb sauce. This sauce is vibrant and refreshing, perfect for adding a burst of flavor to steamed or roasted vegetables. To make this sauce, mix together freshly squeezed lemon juice, high-quality olive oil, and minced garlic. The acidity of the lemon juice brightens up the sauce, while the olive oil adds a rich, smooth texture. Incorporate a variety of chopped fresh herbs such as parsley, basil, and dill, which bring a fresh, aromatic quality to the sauce. Season with a pinch of salt and freshly ground black pepper. This lemon herb sauce can be drizzled over a variety of dishes, from simple steamed asparagus to roasted root vegetables, adding a light and refreshing flavor that enhances the natural taste of the ingredients.

CHAPTER SEVEN

COMFORT FOODS

Classic Comfort Recipes

Classic comfort foods are the heartwarming meals that evoke a sense of nostalgia and home. These dishes, such as beef stew, chicken pot pie, and macaroni and cheese, often remind people of family gatherings and cozy evenings. The beauty of these recipes is that they can be effortlessly prepared in a slow cooker, allowing you to enjoy a delicious, home-cooked meal with minimal effort.

Beef stew is a quintessential comfort food, and making it in a slow cooker enhances its flavors while simplifying the cooking process. To start, choose a cut of beef chuck and cut it into cubes. Searing the beef in a hot skillet before adding it to the slow cooker helps to lock in the flavors and create a rich base for the stew. Next, add a mix of root vegetables—carrots, potatoes, and onions are classic choices. These vegetables not only add depth and texture to the stew but also absorb the savory juices, becoming tender and flavorful. Pour in beef broth until the ingredients are just covered, and season with herbs like thyme and bay leaves. Setting the slow cooker on low for about 8 hours allows the flavors to meld together beautifully, resulting in a hearty, fragrant stew that's perfect for cold evenings. Serve it with a slice of crusty bread to soak up the delicious broth.

Chicken pot pie is another beloved comfort dish that transitions beautifully to the slow cooker. Begin by placing chicken breasts or thighs in the slow cooker. These cuts of chicken are ideal for slow cooking as they remain moist and tender. Add diced potatoes, carrots, and peas to the pot. These vegetables are traditional in pot pie and provide a variety of textures and flavors. Pour in chicken broth to cover the ingredients and season generously with salt, pepper, and thyme. Cooking the mixture on low for 6-7 hours allows the chicken to become tender and the vegetables to soften while absorbing the flavorful broth. Once the cooking time is up, you can create a delightful twist by topping the mixture with a store-bought pie crust or biscuit dough. Transfer the slow cooker insert (if oven-safe) to the oven or use a separate baking dish, and bake until the crust is golden brown. This method combines the ease of slow cooking with the classic finish of a baked pot pie, resulting in a comforting and satisfying meal.

Pasta dishes can be effortlessly transformed into comforting slow cooker meals, making dinner preparation a breeze while infusing the pasta with rich, flavorful ingredients. One of the most beloved options is slow cooker lasagna, a dish that combines the classic flavors of Italian cuisine with the convenience of a slow cooker. To make this, layer uncooked lasagna noodles with a mix of ricotta cheese, marinara sauce, and mozzarella cheese directly in the slow cooker. Start by spreading a thin layer of marinara sauce on the bottom, then add a layer of uncooked noodles. Spread a generous layer of ricotta cheese over the noodles, followed by another layer of marinara sauce and a sprinkling of mozzarella cheese. Repeat these layers until all the ingredients are used, ensuring the top layer is a hearty covering of sauce and cheese. Cover the slow cooker and cook on low for 4-6 hours. During this time, the noodles will cook perfectly, absorbing the savory flavors of the sauce and the creamy richness of the cheeses, resulting in a delightful, cheesy lasagna that's sure to please.

Another fantastic and easy option for slow cooker pasta dishes is slow cooker macaroni and cheese. This classic comfort food becomes even more accessible when made in a slow cooker, requiring minimal effort and delivering maximum flavor. Begin by combining uncooked macaroni, shredded cheddar cheese, milk, and butter in the slow cooker. For an extra layer of flavor, add a touch of mustard, which enhances the cheese's tanginess and adds depth to the dish. Set the slow cooker on low and cook for about 2-3 hours, stirring occasionally to ensure the pasta cooks evenly and the cheese melts smoothly into a creamy sauce. The result is a rich, velvety macaroni and cheese that is sure to be a hit with both kids and adults alike.

Casseroles And One-Pot Meals

Casseroles and one-pot meals are the epitome of comfort food, offering hearty, satisfying dishes with minimal effort. The slow cooker, in particular, is an invaluable tool for creating these meals, as it allows for long, slow cooking that melds flavors beautifully while freeing you from constant kitchen supervision.

A classic example of a slow cooker casserole is chicken and rice. This dish is as simple as it is comforting. Start by placing chicken thighs in the slow cooker. These cuts are perfect for slow cooking due to their higher fat content, which ensures they remain moist and flavorful throughout the long cooking process. Next, add uncooked rice and enough chicken broth to cover the ingredients. The broth not only cooks the rice but also infuses it with rich, savory flavors. To this base, you can add a mix of your favorite vegetables. Broccoli and bell peppers are excellent choices; they add color, texture, and nutritional value to the dish. Season the mixture with garlic powder, onion powder, and pepper to taste. Set your slow cooker to low and let it work its magic for 6-8 hours. The result is a warm, satisfying meal that's ready when you are, with the chicken tender and the rice perfectly cooked and infused with all the flavors of the broth and spices.

Another favorite one-pot meal is slow cooker chili. This dish is perfect for those cold, lazy evenings when you crave something hearty and warming. Start by browning ground beef or turkey in a skillet. Browning the meat before adding it to the slow cooker helps to develop its flavor and improves the overall texture of the chili. Once browned, transfer the meat to the slow cooker. Add canned tomatoes, kidney beans, and your favorite chili spices. Common chili spices include cumin, chili powder, paprika, and a touch of cayenne pepper for some heat. These spices will slowly permeate the chili as it cooks, creating a depth of flavor that's hard to beat. Set the slow cooker to low and let it cook for 6-8 hours. The long, slow cooking process allows the flavors to meld together, resulting in a rich, hearty chili. Serve it with cornbread or over a bed of rice for a complete meal.

Slow Cooker Pizza

Pizza is a beloved comfort food, but making it from scratch can sometimes be a daunting task. Enter the slow cooker—a kitchen appliance that promises to make your pizza preparation both easy and fun. With this method, you can enjoy the deliciousness of pizza without the hassle of traditional baking. Here's how to make a slow cooker pizza that's bound to become a favorite in your household.

Ingredients and Preparation

To start, gather your ingredients: pizza sauce, shredded cheese, and your choice of toppings. Popular options include pepperoni, mushrooms, and bell peppers, but you can get creative with whatever you like. Additionally, you will need pre-made pizza dough, which can be found at most grocery stores or made at home if you prefer.

Begin by preparing your slow cooker. It's a good idea to lightly grease the bottom and sides to prevent sticking. Once that's done, start layering your ingredients. First, pour a generous amount of pizza sauce into the bottom of the slow cooker. Spread it evenly to create a solid base for your pizza. Next, sprinkle a layer of shredded cheese over the sauce. This cheese layer acts as a glue, holding the toppings together and ensuring every bite is cheesy and delightful.

Adding the Toppings

Now it's time to add your chosen toppings. Whether you opt for the classic pepperoni, the earthy mushrooms, or the colorful bell peppers, distribute them evenly over the cheese layer. This step is where you can really personalize your pizza, adding as much or as little of each topping as you desire. Feel free to mix and match toppings to create your perfect pizza combination.

Applying the Dough

Once your toppings are in place, it's time to add the pizza dough. Carefully lay the pre-made dough over the toppings. Press it down gently to ensure it makes contact with all the ingredients underneath. This step is crucial as it allows the dough to absorb the flavors of the sauce and toppings while cooking.

Cooking the Pizza

Set your slow cooker to low and cover it with the lid. Allow the pizza to cook for 3-4 hours. During this time, the dough will rise and cook through, while the cheese will melt and become bubbly. The slow cooker creates a unique cooking environment, resulting in a pizza that is both crispy on the edges and soft in the center.

Finishing Touches

After 3-4 hours, check the pizza to ensure the dough is fully cooked. It should be golden brown on top and cooked through in the center. If it's not quite there yet, give it a little more time. Once done, carefully lift the pizza out of the slow cooker. Let it cool for a few minutes before slicing and serving.

Enjoying Your Creation

This slow cooker pizza offers all the flavors of a traditional pizza with minimal effort. The slow cooking process allows the flavors to meld together beautifully, resulting in a pizza that is both rich and flavorful. It's perfect for busy weeknights, casual gatherings, or any time you want a comforting meal without spending hours in the kitchen.

CHAPTER EIGHT

DESSERTS

Cakes And Puddings

When it comes to desserts, cakes and puddings are classic favorites that can be easily prepared in a slow cooker, providing a delightful end to any meal. Slow cooker cakes, in particular, stand out for their incredibly moist and flavorful texture, benefiting from the gentle, even heat that this cooking method offers. Preparing a slow cooker cake is straightforward and flexible, whether you start with a simple cake mix or make one from scratch. An essential tip is to use a slow cooker liner or generously spray the cooker with non-stick spray to prevent the cake from sticking.

One popular and indulgent recipe is the slow cooker chocolate lava cake. This dessert involves pouring a cake batter into the slow cooker and topping it with a mixture of hot water, sugar, and cocoa powder. As it cooks, the top transforms into a rich, gooey chocolate pudding, while the bottom sets into a moist and tender cake. The result is a decadent, multi-layered dessert that is sure to impress.

Puddings prepared in the slow cooker are equally delightful and comforting. A standout example is bread pudding, a dessert that repurposes stale bread into a delicious treat. To make slow cooker bread pudding, you mix together ingredients like milk, eggs, sugar, and spices with the bread, then pour the mixture into the slow cooker. As it cooks, the pudding sets and develops a golden, slightly crispy top, making for a satisfying dessert that evokes a sense of homey comfort.

Rice pudding is another classic dessert that adapts wonderfully to the slow cooker. Combining rice, milk, sugar, and vanilla, this pudding cooks slowly to create a creamy and satisfying treat. The slow cooker allows the flavors to meld beautifully, resulting in a rich and velvety texture. For added flavor, you can customize your rice pudding by adding raisins, a sprinkle of cinnamon, or even a splash of rum.

Both cakes and puddings benefit greatly from the slow cooker's ability to maintain a consistent, low temperature. This gentle cooking process not only enhances the flavors but also ensures that the desserts remain moist and tender. Whether you're making a cake or a pudding, the slow cooker proves to be a versatile and convenient tool for creating delicious desserts with minimal effort.

Cobblers And Crisps

Cobblers and crisps are ideal desserts for the slow cooker, especially when you have fresh, seasonal fruits to use. These desserts are typically easy to prepare and require minimal effort, making them a convenient choice for busy days or when you want to impress guests without spending hours in the kitchen.

To make a slow cooker cobbler, you can use fruits like peaches, berries, or apples. The first step is to prepare the fruit, which involves washing, peeling (if necessary), and cutting it into bite-sized pieces. Once the fruit is ready, mix it with sugar and a bit of lemon juice to enhance the flavor and help the fruit release its juices as it cooks. The fruit mixture is then spread evenly in the bottom of the slow cooker.

Next, prepare the batter for the cobbler topping. This simple batter is made from common pantry ingredients: flour, sugar, baking powder, and milk. Some recipes might also include a pinch of salt or a bit of melted butter to add richness. Once the batter is mixed until smooth, it is poured over the fruit in the slow cooker. As the cobbler cooks, the batter will rise and form a cake-like topping over the sweet, bubbly fruit, creating a delicious contrast in texture.

Crisps, on the other hand, have a crumbly topping made from oats, flour, sugar, and butter. To make an apple crisp in the slow cooker, start by slicing apples and mixing them with sugar and cinnamon. The cinnamon adds a warm, spicy note that pairs beautifully with the apples. Once the apples are evenly coated with the sugar and cinnamon mixture, they are placed in the slow cooker.

The topping for the crisp is made by combining oats, flour, sugar, and butter. The butter should be cold and cut into small pieces so that it can be worked into the dry ingredients, creating a crumbly texture. Some recipes might also include nuts or spices like nutmeg for extra flavor. The oat mixture is then sprinkled over the apples in the slow cooker. As the crisp cooks, the apples become tender and juicy while the topping turns golden and crunchy, creating a delightful combination of textures and flavors.

Custards And Flans

Custards and flans are creamy desserts that can be exquisitely cooked in a slow cooker, achieving a perfect texture through the appliance's gentle heat. These desserts rely on a precise balance of eggs, sugar, and milk or cream, and the slow cooker's steady temperature helps prevent curdling and overcooking, common pitfalls when using traditional oven methods.

Classic Vanilla Custard

A classic vanilla custard, for instance, is made by whisking together eggs, sugar, and milk. This mixture is then poured into individual ramekins. To ensure even cooking, these ramekins are placed in the slow cooker with a bit of water, creating a bain-marie, or water bath. This method of indirect heat cooking is ideal for custards, as it allows the dessert to set slowly and evenly without the risk of scorching or curdling. The result is a smooth, silky custard that can be enhanced with various flavors, such as vanilla, chocolate, or coffee.

The slow cooker's gentle heat ensures that the eggs in the custard cook slowly, forming a creamy and luscious texture. The bain-marie is crucial as it provides a moist cooking environment, preventing the custard from drying out or developing a rubbery texture. Once cooked, the custards can be chilled and served with a sprinkle of nutmeg, a drizzle of caramel, or a garnish of fresh fruit.

Caramel Flan

Flans are similar to custards but often include a caramel layer, adding a delightful sweetness and a touch of elegance to the dessert. To make a caramel flan, sugar is first cooked until it turns a rich golden brown, transforming into caramel. This caramel is then poured into the bottom of a mold. The egg, sugar, and milk mixture is poured over the caramel, and the entire mold is placed in the slow cooker.

As with custards, the slow cooker's gentle heat cooks the flan evenly, allowing the flavors to meld beautifully. The flan is ready when it is set and has a slight jiggle in the center. After cooling, the mold is inverted onto a serving plate, revealing the luscious caramel topping that cascades over the flan.

Benefits of Slow Cooker Desserts

Using a slow cooker for these desserts offers several benefits. The even and low temperature reduces the risk of overcooking, and the bain-marie method keeps the desserts moist. Additionally, the slow cooker is a hands-off appliance, freeing up the cook to focus on other tasks or simply relax while the desserts slowly come to perfection.

Sweet Bread And Roll Recipes

Sweet breads and rolls can be delightful additions to any meal, and using a slow cooker to bake them can yield soft, flavorful treats that are hard to resist. The slow, steady heat of a slow cooker helps maintain moisture and ensures an even bake, making it an excellent method for creating delicious baked goods without the need for a traditional oven. Let's explore two popular recipes: cinnamon roll bread and banana bread.

One of the most beloved sweet bread recipes is cinnamon roll bread. This recipe begins with a basic bread dough, which you can prepare using flour, yeast, sugar, milk, and butter. Once the dough has risen, roll it out into a rectangular shape. Then, generously spread softened butter over the surface of the dough. Sprinkle a mixture of cinnamon and sugar evenly over the butter. The next step is to roll the dough up tightly, starting from one of the longer sides, to form a log. Slice the log into individual rolls, about one to two inches thick. Place these rolls into the slow cooker, allowing enough space between them for expansion as they rise.

As the rolls cook slowly, they become incredibly soft and gooey. The slow cooker's gentle heat ensures that the cinnamon and sugar melt into the dough, creating a luscious, caramelized filling. This method results in rolls that are perfect for a special breakfast or a delectable dessert. For an added touch of indulgence, you can drizzle the warm rolls with a simple icing made from powdered sugar and milk once they're done baking.

Another fantastic sweet bread recipe suited for the slow cooker is banana bread. Start by mashing ripe bananas and mixing them with flour, sugar, eggs, and a bit of baking soda. This combination creates a thick batter that transforms into a moist, flavorful loaf as it cooks. The slow cooker's even heat distribution ensures that the banana bread bakes uniformly without drying out, resulting in a perfect texture.

The beauty of banana bread lies in its versatility. You can customize it by adding a variety of mix-ins such as chopped nuts, chocolate chips, or dried fruit. These additions can enhance the flavor and texture, making each loaf unique and personalized. Simply pour the prepared batter into a greased slow cooker and let it cook until the bread is set and a toothpick inserted into the center comes out clean.

CHAPTER NINE

TIPS AND TRICKS FOR SUCCESS

Time-Saving Tips

Cooking with a slow cooker is all about convenience, and there are several ways to make it even more efficient. One of the best time-saving tips is to prepare your ingredients the night before. Chop vegetables, marinate meats, and measure out spices ahead of time. In the morning, simply place everything in the slow cooker, set the timer, and go about your day. This method not only saves time in the morning rush but also ensures that all your ingredients are well-prepared and ready to go.

Another great tip is to use slow cooker liners. These disposable bags fit inside your slow cooker and make cleanup a breeze.

Once your meal is finished, just remove the liner and throw it away. This saves you from scrubbing stubborn, stuck-on food from the pot, allowing you to enjoy your meal without dreading the cleanup. Slow cooker liners are especially useful when cooking dishes that tend to leave a residue or when you're short on time and can't deal with extensive cleaning.

Consider investing in a programmable slow cooker. These models allow you to set specific cooking times and temperatures, and they often switch to a "keep warm" mode once the cooking time is complete. This feature ensures your meal is ready when you are, without overcooking. Programmable slow cookers are perfect for busy individuals who might not be home to turn off the cooker at the right time. The keep warm feature also means your food stays at a safe, warm temperature until you're ready to eat.

Batch cooking is another excellent time-saving strategy. Prepare large quantities of slow cooker meals and freeze portions for later use. This way, you only need to cook once but can enjoy multiple meals. When you're ready to eat, simply thaw and reheat. This approach is particularly beneficial for those with hectic schedules who may not have time to cook every day. Batch cooking also allows for more efficient use of ingredients, reducing food waste.

Additionally, choosing recipes with minimal prep work can save time. Look for slow cooker meals that require little to no pre-cooking or chopping. Recipes that call for whole or large pieces of vegetables and meats can be just as delicious with less effort. These recipes are perfect for days when you're particularly pressed for time but still want a home-cooked meal.

Using the right tools can also streamline your slow cooker experience. For example, a good set of kitchen knives can make chopping vegetables faster and easier. Measuring cups and spoons ensure you add the right amount of spices and liquids, which can save you from making corrections later. Having a dedicated space in your kitchen for slow cooker prep can also make the process more efficient. Keep your slow cooker, liners, utensils, and frequently used ingredients in one area to minimize the time spent searching for items.

Finally, don't be afraid to experiment with different cooking times and settings. Understanding how your slow cooker works best with various recipes can help you optimize your cooking process. Some meals might cook better on high for a shorter period, while others are best on low for several hours. Experimentation can lead to discovering the most efficient and delicious ways to use your slow cooker.

Enhancing Flavors In Slow Cooking

Slow cooking is an excellent method for developing deep, rich flavors in your dishes, but there are several techniques you can employ to elevate these flavors even further. One of the most effective strategies is to brown your meat before adding it to the slow cooker. Searing meat on the stovetop caramelizes the exterior, creating a complex layer of flavor that enhances the overall dish. This Maillard reaction not only adds depth but also imparts a savory richness that can't be replicated through slow cooking alone.

In addition to browning meat, the order in which you layer your ingredients is crucial for maximizing flavor. Begin by placing root vegetables, such as carrots and potatoes, along with tougher cuts of meat at the bottom of the slow cooker. This placement is strategic, as these ingredients will be exposed to the most heat, allowing them to soften and infuse their flavors into the broth. On the other hand, more delicate vegetables and fresh herbs should be added later in the cooking process. This prevents them from becoming overly mushy and allows them to retain their vibrant flavors and textures.

Another essential aspect of enhancing flavors is the use of aromatic ingredients. Garlic and onions are fundamental to many recipes, providing a fragrant base that complements a wide range of dishes. Fresh herbs, such as rosemary and thyme, also play a vital role in flavor enhancement. Their aromatic oils release into the dish during the slow cooking process, imparting a wonderful fragrance and taste. For an even greater impact, consider adding a bouquet garni or herb sachet, which allows for easy removal of herbs while still infusing your dish with their flavors.

Finally, don't underestimate the power of acidity in your slow-cooked meals. Adding a splash of acid—like vinegar or citrus juice—towards the end of cooking can significantly brighten the overall flavor profile. Acidity helps to balance the richness of the ingredients, enhancing the taste and making each bite more enjoyable. This simple step can elevate a good dish to an exceptional one, providing a delightful contrast that excites the palate.

Adapting Traditional Recipes For Slow Cooking

Slow cooking has become a popular method for preparing meals, allowing for deeper flavors and tender textures without the constant attention that stovetop cooking requires. Adapting traditional recipes for the slow cooker can be a rewarding way to enjoy familiar dishes with a twist. Here's how to make those adjustments effectively.

Liquid Reduction

One of the primary considerations when adapting a recipe is the liquid content. Traditional cooking methods often call for generous amounts of broth, water, or wine. However, slow cookers are designed to trap moisture, meaning that excess liquid can lead to a watery dish. As a rule of thumb, reduce the amount of liquid by about half. This adjustment will help achieve the right consistency while still allowing for the absorption of flavors.

Cooking Times and Temperatures

The next step is adjusting cooking times and temperatures to suit the slow cooker's unique settings. Generally, the high setting on a slow cooker mimics an oven temperature of around 300 degrees

Fahrenheit, while the low setting is equivalent to approximately 200 degrees. For recipes that typically require 30 minutes to 1 hour in the oven, you can expect them to need about 4 to 6 hours on high or 8 to 10 hours on low in a slow cooker. This extended cooking time allows for the flavors to meld beautifully and ensures that tougher cuts of meat become tender.

Dairy Products and Starches

Another important consideration is the timing of dairy products. Milk, cheese, and cream can curdle if subjected to prolonged cooking times. To avoid this issue, add these ingredients during the last 30 minutes of cooking. This ensures that they retain their creamy texture and flavor without compromising the dish.

When it comes to starches like pasta and rice, their quick cooking times can pose a challenge in the slow cooker. If added too early, they can become overcooked and mushy. A better approach is to cook these ingredients separately and incorporate them into the dish just before serving. This not only maintains their texture but also allows you to control their doneness more effectively.

Cleaning And Maintaining Your Slow Cooker

Proper care of your slow cooker is essential for its longevity and performance, allowing you to enjoy delicious meals for years to come. The cleaning process is straightforward, but it requires a bit of attention to detail to ensure that all components are well-maintained.

Begin by unplugging your slow cooker and allowing it to cool completely before starting the cleaning process. This safety measure not only protects you from burns but also prevents damage to the appliance. Once cooled, carefully remove the stoneware insert. This part can be washed using warm, soapy water. When cleaning, opt for a soft sponge or cloth to avoid scratching the insert's surface, as abrasive materials can cause unsightly damage.

If you find stubborn, stuck-on food remnants after a cooking session, don't worry. A simple soaking solution can work wonders. Fill the insert with warm, soapy water and allow it to soak for a few hours or even overnight. This will help loosen any residue, making it easier to wash away. For particularly tough spots, you can create a paste using baking soda and water. Gently scrub the affected areas with this paste, ensuring you don't scratch the surface.

While the insert is the most frequently used component, the exterior of the slow cooker also requires attention. Wipe down the outside with a damp cloth, taking care to avoid immersing the base in water. Excess moisture can damage electrical components, so it's crucial to keep the base dry.

Regular maintenance includes checking the power cord for any signs of wear or damage. If you notice fraying or other issues, replace the cord immediately to ensure safe operation.

For a deeper clean, consider running a periodic maintenance cycle. To do this, fill the stoneware insert with a mixture of water, white vinegar, and baking soda. Turn your slow cooker to the high setting and let it run for a few hours. This mixture will not only clean but also help eliminate any lingering odors and stains, leaving your slow cooker fresh and ready for your next culinary adventure.

THE END